Need a Stress-less Moment?

Massage

The Ultimate Stress Reliever

Herbert Gooden

CMT, NMT, CRC Instructor

Published by Herbert Gooden II

Birmingham, Alabama

Need a Stress – Less Moment?

Massage

The Ultimate Stress Reliever

Published by Herbert Gooden II

Birmingham, Alabama

Copyright © 2013 by Herbert Gooden.

Cover by Ahtsham Iqbal Alvi

Edited by Cory Emberson

This publication is not intended as a substitute for the advice of a health care professionals.

Stress-Less-Moments.MassageTherapy.com

ISBN 10:1-4942-7989-4
ISBN 13: 978-1-4942-7989-9
PRODUCED IN THE UNITED STATES OF AMERICA

About the Author

Herbert Gooden is a graduate of the Red Mountain Institute for the Healing Arts in Birmingham, Alabama, and is trained in Clinical Massage Therapy. He is a Clinical and Neuromuscular Massage Therapist at Ross Bridge Golf and Spa Resort and has provided therapeutic massage services to more than ten thousand clients. His passion is being involved in the healing ministry through massage, as well as allowing others to pause in their daily life to take care of themselves so they can take care of each other.

He has worked with many clients in multiple forms of clinical massage to relieve stress, including Swedish, deep tissue, Thai yoga, prenatal massage, repetitive use injury therapy, and more. He has spent more than twenty years studying and teaching groups and individuals in personal and spiritual development.

Beyond his work at Ross Bridge Golf and Spa Resort, he also provides therapeutic massages for employees at Children's of Alabama Hospital. He aspires to continue his research in the healing arts through massage, and his passion continues to grow as the field continues to grow as well. His hope is for others to receive a massage and have an experience that will benefit them long after their treatment session.

Dedication

This book is dedicated to my wife Tanya and the thousands of clients who have allowed me to share and grow with them, as I serve my fellow man through the power of touch.

CONTENTS

About the Author..*iii*

Dedication ....*iv*

Introduction 1

Chapter 1: What is Stress? 7

   Good or Bad Stress? 7

Chapter 2: What is Cortisol Poisoning?.............11

   Which Body Systems Can Be Damaged

   by Excessive Stress?.......................................11

Chapter 3: What are Alpha Waves? 17

   What is the Alpha State? 17

Chapter 4: What is Mindfulness? 19

   What are the Benefits of Mindfulness?..................19

   How to Practice Mindfulness 21

   How to Practice Meditation................................23

Chapter 5: What is a Therapeutic Body

Massage? 27

   What is a Massage? 27

   What are the Physical Benefits of Massage? 28

   What are the Chemical and Mental Benefits

   of Massage? 29

   What are the Spiritual Benefits of Massage? 30

   Get a Massage! Your Spirit Will Never be

   the Same!..33

Chapter 6: Where Do I Start? 35

   How to Find a Licensed Massage Therapist........35

   What to Expect Before, During, and After

   Your Massage 38

   Appendix A: Autogenic Relaxation Training 43

Appendix B: Long Form Meditation 49
Appendix C: More Healthful Massage Benefits 55
Testimonials..57

Introduction

You have been working a long time to get to this point—stressed! There was a time when you were relaxed, peaceful, happy, and full of joy, with not a care in the world ... looking forward to the day before you. Wow, has that changed. Over the years as you have grown into adulthood, layers of stressful events and situations have come into your life. You are not at ease as often as you would like to be. Your joy has turned into feeling like a nervous wreck. You find yourself constantly feeling tightness in your stomach area or tension in your head. You sometimes find yourself viewing life in a pessimistic way. Sometimes you may feel stuck and unable to move forward.

Stress has become a way of life in this modern world, and you are part of this modern world. Medical studies report that 80% to 90% of all disease is stress-related. Unless you learn to do something about it, the pressures of life and the damage to your body caused by stress will push you six feet under prematurely.

Can you imagine having a day with less stress? How would you like to have a day where your mind and body were in a harmonized state of peace, and open and receptive to any situation without reacting to it in a negative way? I know that it seems out of reach because of how you are feeling now. I know how you feel—I have been there before. In the past, I have let daily life challenges get me so out of whack that I ended up in the hospital and close to being six feet under, literally. I had let family pressures, job pressures, and relationships get the better of me. I just could not live life on life's terms.

Pain, suffering, sickness, and death all can result from excessive stress. There is a road to the peace and serenity you deserve. There is a way not only to get stress relief, but a tool that I will present to you will also help you manage it. This information is simple and straightforward. You will have to make a small contribution of effort in order to receive the full benefits, but the majority of the time you only have a passive role to play. You will receive some additional tools that you can utilize to help you prepare for the ultimate passive tool for stress relief. The additional tools can be used before or after your treatment. If used before your treatment, they will give you an idea of how you will feel during treatment. When these tools are used afterward, they will be a resource to have and use to help maintain stress relief between your treatments.

These steps have been carefully designed to take you from where you are to where you want to be, from a life of stress and confusion to a life with more moments of peace and serenity. There are many ways and attempts out there in the world to treat stress. Some try to treat stress through the body with exercise, and some through the mind with drugs. There is a lot of confusion as to what stress is and how to treat it. Here are six myths that surround stress. Dispelling them enables us to understand our problems and then take action against them. Let's look at these myths.

Myth 1: Stress is the same for everybody.

Completely wrong. Stress is different for each of us. What is stressful for one person may or may not be stressful for another; each of us responds to stress in an entirely different way.

Myth 2: Stress is always bad for you.

According to this view, zero stress makes us happy and healthy. Wrong. Stress is to the human condition what tension is to the violin string—too little and the music is dull and raspy; too much and the music is shrill or the string snaps. Stress can be the kiss of death or the spice of life. The issue, really, is how to manage it. Managed stress makes us productive and happy; mismanaged stress hurts and even kills us.

Myth 3: Stress is everywhere, so you can't do anything about it.

Not so. You can plan your life so that stress does not overwhelm you. Effective planning involves setting priorities and working on simple problems first, solving them, and then going on to more complex difficulties. When stress is mismanaged, it's difficult to prioritize. All your problems seem to be equal, and stress seems to be everywhere.

Myth 4: The most popular techniques for reducing stress are the best ones.

Again, not so. No universally effective stress reduction techniques exist. We are all different, our lives are different, our situations are different, and our reactions are different. Only a comprehensive program tailored to the individual works.

Myth 5: No symptoms, no stress.

Absence of symptoms does not mean the absence of stress. In fact, camouflaging symptoms with medication may deprive you of the signals you need to reduce the strain on your physiological and psychological systems.

Myth 6: Only major symptoms of stress require attention.

This myth assumes that the "minor" symptoms, such as headaches or heartburn, may be safely ignored. Minor symptoms of stress are the early warnings that your life is getting out of hand and that you need to do a better job of managing stress.

When we react to stress, it affects both our mind and our body. This is sometimes referred to as the mind-body experience. Chapter 1 defines stress and the effects it has on our body, both good and bad. You may ask yourself: Is there good stress? Yes, there is, and we will show you how to differentiate it from the bad stressors. Chapter 2 explains and describes how our bodies can poison themselves from too much stress.

As you move on to Chapter 3, you will gain knowledge about alpha waves and the alpha state, which is the primary goal of the exercises found in the chapter immediately following it, as well as therapeutic massage. Something magical happens when we are in the alpha state. In Chapter 4, you will begin to learn how to use two great and simple tools: awareness and meditation. Both tools can be used before and after your treatment to begin the process or maintain the feeling of relaxation. Chapter 5 is where you will be introduced to what I feel is the greatest passive tool discovered in the past few thousand years: massage. In that chapter, you will gain knowledge about therapeutic massages and the physical, chemical, mental, and the spiritual benefits you will receive. Chapter 6 shows you how to begin the process of finding and selecting a Licensed Massage Therapist. This chapter also helps you to know beforehand what you should expect, before, during, and after a massage.

You may want to go directly to the exercises found in Chapter 4 or after reading Chapter 5, go out and get a massage. This process works with or without the knowledge of what is happening in the background to your body and mind when you are under damage causing stress. You can refer back to Chapters 1 and 2 if you would like to know what's going on in the background when you are in stressful situations. The appendix contains a wealth of valuable information to help you relax on your own time.

I practice these exercises on a regular basis, and I receive a massage once a week. I believe in these tools and receiving massages as a highly effective way to relieve stress and to manage it. I believe in this to the point that after 22-plus years in communications and design, and serving as Head of Operations, that I changed careers and became a Certified Massage Therapist and Instructor. This is tried and tested information. It works. I am a facilitator and witness to the thousands who have benefited after taking these steps. So join me on this journey that will literally change your life and restore some **calm** into it.

Chapter 1
What is Stress?

Good or Bad Stress?

Herbert! I was just in an ugly dispute, and I am stressed out! I just got a speeding ticket, and I am stressed out! My boss just told me to meet the deadline or I will be demoted—I am so stressed out! My kids are acting so terrible—I am *so* stressed!

These are just a few examples of the many statements that my clients make when they come in for a massage. They are breathing very rapidly and appear very anxious. They begin to tell their story and are very animated when telling me why they are feeling stressed. As they continue to tell their story, they point to or identify where they feel the stress in their bodies. Some say it feels all tight in their head. Others name different anatomical parts of their body where they feel the tension is or effects of the stress.

In modern times, stress receives a front seat in our lives as it relates to our mental and physical health. Experts estimate that 80% to 90% of disease is stress related. There are numerous books and articles about stress syndromes, stress personalities, and stressful environments. We have entire institutions that are devoted to the study of stress. There are workshops and clinics teaching us how to recognize stress, how to avoid it, or how to reduce it. There are also workshops on how to recover from it, cope with it, or how to live with it.

We all experience stress on a day-to-day basis. Some of us have had challenges that cause us to tense up or make us feel uncomfortable in some way. Sometimes our minds feel as though there is someone inside, tightening down screws or bolts. It sometimes makes us feel anxious, exhausted, or helpless. Its victims are male and female, and it crosses all nationalities and ages. What is this term **stress,** which is uttered so often when our body and mental faculties are challenged?

One of Merriam-Webster's Dictionary's meanings for stress is "a physical, chemical, or emotional factor that causes bodily or mental tension and may be a factor in disease causation." This definition is quite suitable for the way we humans react to outside stimuli that we encounter on a day-to-day basis.

We humans are equipped with a **stress response system**. Big reactions to big threats, and small reactions to small threats are signs of a healthy stress response system. This response system is the link between the central nervous system and the endocrine system. This system allows us to respond to both short-term and long-term stressors. It is controlled by the hypothalamus-pituitary-adrenal axis (HPA): the communication between the hypothalamus, the pituitary gland, and the adrenals. A **stressor** is a chemical or biological agent, environmental condition, external stimulus, or an event that causes stress to an organism.

Some common stressors that may trigger the response system are loud noises, too much light, lost items, quality and quantity of physical exercise, job demand versus job control, divorce, death, tobacco and alcohol, and societal and family demands. The chemical changes that are brought about when a threat is perceived, and then neutralized once the threat has passed, is a sure sign of a properly functioning stress response system. Just imagine a unit of soldiers being threatened and attacked by enemy troops. They defend and defeat and go back to their normal operational activity that existed before the threat.

The paradox to any of the stressors before mentioned is how we perceive the event taking place. You can be in a distressing situation that you cannot alter, avoid, or accept. Psychologist Richard Lazarus coined the term "Eustress," which is stress with a positive effect. Within my private practice, work-related stress is a common complaint. One example would be a demanding boss who requires you to perform at a level beyond what you think is possible. Another constant stressor is strained personal relationships. This could be perceived as threat or as a challenge. However, with the right mental resources, how we view any given situation has the possibility to be perceived as a challenge instead of a threat. This means that it could be approached with enthusiasm instead of dread.

There is a chemical difference that is essential to understanding how the brain functions when it perceives an event as a healthy challenge or a threat. If the event is perceived as good (stress), it should mobilize and motivate us. If the event is bad (stress), it overwhelms, paralyzes, or demoralizes us.

When our energy is high and we are in a positive mood, the sympathetic nervous system is activated, and the adrenal glands secrete chemicals called **catecholamines.** The catecholamines, adrenaline and noradrenalin, arouse us to action in a more productive way. We look at the situation and think how we may handle it. But when the brain goes into emergency mode (fight or flight), it starts pumping **cortisol.** It has been shown that boredom, impatience, frustration, and even tiredness have also caused an increase in cortisol.

Cortisol results from an elevated level of catecholamine. It is a steroid hormone and one of a group of glucocorticoids secreted by adrenal cortex; it influences the metabolism of proteins. It is the hormone secreted under long-term, low-grade stress and is measurable in the saliva. Cortisol is important for several reasons. It is a very powerful anti-inflammatory and is sometimes used systemically or locally for that purpose. Problems begin when its level is elevated and is secreted for a prolonged period within our body systems.

Remember the soldiers mentioned earlier? The troops would continue to fight and use unnecessary energy although the enemy was defeated. In other words, they would begin to fight with each other, destroying themselves. This is what happens when cortisol is released at an elevated level and begins to poison the human body.

Chapter 2
What is Cortisol Poisoning?

Which Body Systems Can Be Damaged by Excessive Stress?

The biochemical effects of the secretion of the hypothalamus, the pituitary gland, and adrenals play their part in the preparation of the nervous system, the muscles, and the organs for handling injury, a threat, or an emergency. They prepare the body and the mind so we can respond to take flight or fight, or whatever is necessary to prevent harm to ourselves. Example: You see a freight train heading directly toward you; you jump out of the way instinctively and without thought. This is the system working and calling you to a healthy response.

The problem starts when the levels of these hormones are introduced to the bloodstream for a sustained period of time. This occurs when repeated episodes of stress takes place. When this takes place, very different changes occur in the nervous system and other target tissue. The hormones involved in this occurrence have a pharmacological effect on the target tissue. Pharmacological effects can be therapeutic, toxic, or lethal. The term "therapeutic effect" describes a situation whereby a drug successfully treats a given condition. Toxicity, on the other hand, results from harmful pharmacological effects. Lethal (deadly) effects are often related to dosage. One common pharmacological effect is the inhibition of inflammation around injuries or infections. This is essentially why large doses of cortisol—or its synthetic, cortisone—are administered in cases where the infections, allergies, arthritis, and similar inflammatory conditions have reached a dangerous level.

Inflammation in most cases is of great value and a normal response to injury. This is how the body floods the area with oxygen, nutrients, antibodies to fight off invading organisms, and fibroblasts to carry on the wound-healing processes to the injured area. However, you may see how sustained levels of cortisol in the bloodstream may actually interfere with the natural healing process and progressively decrease the body's resistance to infections, swelling, and tumors of all kinds.

Adrenaline, the same compound that is secreted by the nerve ends of the sympathetic branch of the autonomic nervous system, has an important pharmacological effect as opposed to its main biochemical ones. As long as adrenaline is secreted, it prevents its target organs from entering a phase of rest and recovery. When this takes place, the effect upon your bodily organs is as if you have not had enough sleep or are so exhausted that they become dysfunctional.

Sustained high levels of adrenaline and cortisol suppress healthy inflammation and the autonomic nervous system. The excessive increase can cause high blood pressure, gastric ulceration, and atherosclerosis, suppression of the immune system (which would lower one's resistance to disease and infections of all kinds), sterility, and significant personality changes.

You may ask yourself, are these not the same chemicals that are released in my body in order to safeguard it during an emergency? Have you ever heard of "too much of a good thing"? Chronic stress, or frequently recurring stress, creates a kind of adrenaline/cortisol poisoning. This is similar to the way in which repeated doses of cocaine or heroin eventually destroys and causes physical and psychological damage to the original beneficial pain-relieving effects.

There is extensive documented evidence on the chemistry and the physiology of stress and how we learn to be sick. There are examples that explain how we can develop a lust after the very things that trigger a system within us that can destroy us. The stimulants that converge on the hypothalamus and the effects produced by an alarm are very complex. The events that take place in our lives vary, and what is perceived by one to be a threat may be perceived as a healthy challenge to another. This implies that we learn to overdose ourselves with adrenaline and cortisol. When we overdose our bodies, our bodies become accustom to the conditions imposed by chronic stress. There are some unique and dangerous things that take place as we adapt.

Changes that take place in the development of the pituitary/adrenal axis equally worsen conditions and limitations on our adaptability. In reality, the total absence of stressful stimulation is not healthier for the development of our adaptive behavior than too much stress. Part of our adaptive healthy development needs an optimal level of stress. In order for the physical and mental faculties to fully develop and assert themselves, a favorable level of adrenal secretion must be released into the bloodstream. The normal operation of our hypothalamus/pituitary/adrenal system, which does include at times full-scale alert, is a necessary element for healthy growth of the body's tissue. One of the essentials of normal growth and function of these precious nerves and glands is adequate **tactile stimulation.**

Experiments have shown that laboratory animals that were held or stimulated in their infancy at various times elicited a healthy pituitary/adrenal response. They quickly achieved high blood levels of stress hormones, and when the threat disappeared, these levels drop just as quickly. But the non-stimulated animals achieved these same blood levels of stress hormones much more slowly, and these high levels are maintained for a much longer time after the threat has been removed. Our response to stress is whether our system responds appropriately and normally to feed it and strengthen it, or inappropriate and abnormally to weaken it.

As we begin to understand the possibilities and importance of bodywork, we begin to see that adequate tactile stimulation, or touch, has a major role in establishing and maintaining the healthy glandular response that trigger the beginning and appropriate withdrawal of the stress hormones. One very potent and beneficial effect of tactile stimulation is the heightening of sensory **awareness**. This awareness can create an early warning system for the beginning of stressful situations. This opens us up to the possibilities of cultivating habits and states of mind that can also help us in our reactions to stress. Before we go into therapeutic massage and its many benefits, let's take a look at mindful awareness and some techniques that you can learn in order to raise your level of mindful awareness.

Chapter 3
What are Alpha Waves?

What is the Alpha State?

You may be asking, Herbert, why do I need to know about alpha waves or the alpha state? Scientific research has shown, with the help of biofeedback equipment, that good things happen to the body when the brain is at the alpha level. Organs and stressed systems recuperate and become revitalized.

You have experienced the alpha state numerous times in your life. It is the natural, comfortable, peaceful, and relaxed state that we pass through on our way to sleep at night and upon awakening in the morning. Alpha waves are present in the brain at different stages of the wake-sleep cycle. The alpha waves rhythms are 8–13 cycles per second.

The most widely researched is during the relaxed mental state, when the subject is at rest with eyes closed, but is not tired or asleep. The subject becomes very relaxed. Good things happen to the body when the brain is at the alpha level. When you are in the alpha state, some of the physiological changes that occur in the body are slowed heart rate and respiratory rate, with the direct result that the body's use of oxygen and production of carbon dioxide drops, indicating an overall reduction in the rate of metabolism. You also gain control of formerly uncontrollable functions. These are just a few examples of what takes place in your body and mind when you are in the alpha state, which occurs when you utilize the exercises found in Chapter 4 or receive a therapeutic massage.

Chapter 4
What is Mindfulness?

What are the Benefits of Mindfulness?

Throughout the scientific community, studies have confirmed that the practice of mindfulness can calm and balance the mind. **Mindfulness is a moment-by-moment awareness.** It can aid us in relating to difficulties and seemingly threatening experiences that cause stress. Mindfulness is awareness without absorption in our thought processes. It is always in the present moment.

One of the mindfulness exercises that I sometimes guide my first-time clients through, because of their nervousness about getting a massage, is what I call the "follow my hands exercise." I instruct the client to focus on my hands and their movements. I ask them to pay attention to the speed and the pressures that I apply. I also ask them to inform me if I need to adjust the speed or pressure that I am exerting.

This simple mindfulness exercise produces a very calming effect within the client. You will notice in this simple exercise a call to pay attention is required, which is also a part of the mindfulness process. By asking my client to participate in this simple exercise, their pre-massage nervousness melts away. As you can see by this example, mindfulness allows us to be less reactive to what is happening in the moment.

To recognize what is happening in the present moment is to be mindful and awake. The opposite of mindfulness is mindlessness. Have you ever forgotten a person's name as soon as you heard it? Have you ever smacked chewing gum so loudly that someone had to tell you to stop? Have you ever completed a task and didn't remember doing it? These are just a few examples of mindlessness. One mindlessness action that causes us more stress than practically any other act is when we allow our minds to be preoccupied with something that has happened in the past or some type of fear about the future, both of which can cause us to suffer.

In order to have calm about the present, we have to be present and not judge or reject what is happening at the moment. This is not only energizing, but it can also allow us to have a clear head. It can also bring some calm to the event that is causing us stress. If we want an experience to be different than it is, awareness will not occur. Your intention must be directed somewhere.

As you consistently return to the present moment, it will begin to have a continual, cumulative effect over time. When you are practicing mindfulness, you are not detaching but actually bringing the mind and body into a more intimate relationship. It is difficult to put these experiences into words, because awareness happens before words arise. In your practice, mindfulness exercises will become subtler or lighter to your perception. Each moment of mindfulness will free you from those stressful moments.

You may wonder why I am explaining what awareness is and the practice of mindfulness. This state of being aware is easily produced with massage. When you combine mindfulness and massage, you will have two resources that are proven to reduce stress. Mindfulness could be a prerequisite to massage, and massage could allow you to know how it feels to be aware. Win, Win, Win.

How to Practice Mindfulness

Mindfulness means being fully aware of everything that's happening, without being emotionally involved. The mindfulness technique allows you to practice "full awareness without emotions" in the quiet time of meditation so that you can carry this awareness into every activity in life.

Mindfulness is a practice that has to be experienced to be understood. There are different levels of practice and intensity. You can perform simple exercise throughout the day such as stopping what you are actively doing and just take a deep breath. Once you stop, you could ask yourself, "How do I feel right now? Am I aware of what I am doing right now? Am I tense or relaxed?" We can do this as often as we need to throughout our day. Below you will find some simple mindfulness exercises. After these exercises, we will explore **meditation,** a slightly more advanced form of mindfulness.

Exercise 1

Stop whatever activity you are involved in. You can stand or sit. Become aware and focus on your breathing. Take a few seconds or a few minutes and experience the sensations in your body. How are you feeling? What do you observe is happening? Don't try to change what you observe or feel—just continue to breathe. Just continue to focus on the *now*. Remember you are not trying to make anything different, you are just observing. Accept this moment just as it is, not as you would like it to be. In your mind and in your heart, feel and know that it's okay in this moment. After a period of time when you are ready, mindfully and with resolve move in the direction your mind tells you to go.

Exercise 2

Stop whatever you are doing. Ask yourself, "Am I awake?" "Am I aware?" "What is on my mind?" or, "What am I thinking right now?"

Exercise 3

Taking in a full breath, notice it as it comes in and fills your lungs. Now breathe out, keeping your mind just on the breath as you exhale. Put out of your mind all ideas except your breath. Do not think about your next activity, whether it be mental or physical, outside of focusing on your breath. If your mind begins to wander, return your thought to your breath. Continue to practice this exercise during reading, walking, or any simple task that will allow you without distractions. With practice, you will be able to tie strings of awareness moments together.

These are just a few simple mindful exercises. As you practice these, you will begin experiencing a subtle peace. There are many books written pertaining to this subject. Hopefully, this will inspire you to seek out other resources.

Now, let's look at another advanced form of mindfulness: meditation.

How to Practice Meditation

Meditation is seeing things more clearly. It is mindfulness directed and extended over a longer period of time. If we are living, we are going to experience some form of stress. Stress is inherent to the human condition. We do not have to be a victim to every stressful situation that arises. Meditation is another tool that allows you to work through some of your stressful situations, understand them, and find meaning in them. If practiced consistently, meditation has a way of allowing us to view stressful situations differently and use that energy to grow in strength, wisdom, and compassion.

Our minds are similar to a standing and undisturbed pond when relaxed. The surface is smooth and calm, and you can see clearly down to the bottom. But throw or skip a rock (stress) across it, and a ripple is produced across the surface. The wave of the ripple is determined by the size of the rock or stone and the amount of forced applied when it was thrown. Our minds unlike the pond, which will settle back down after the stones have taken their course, will continue to produce the ripples effect, long after the stress has been removed.

The practice of meditation gives us a tool that not only prepares us for stress but offers us a method that we can utilize when stress arises. One of my favorite practices that anyone with a little patience can learn is to choose a word or short phrase that has a positive and affirming meaning or feeling to you. When you think of this word it should evoke, love, peace, patience, hope, faith, gentleness, joy, kindness, goodness, and so on.

This technique is simple to learn and use. This may not respond as fast as Mother Nature's fight-or-flight system, which is needed in an emergency situation. However, you can call on it, and there is a high probability that you have triggered it unknowingly. And as with any new skill, the more you practice and apply it to your daily situations, the more you will experience the magic of it working.

There are two simple steps: First, repeat a word, a sound, a prayer, or a phrase that evokes a feeling of, love, peace, patience, hope, faith, gentleness, joy, kindness, or goodness. Second: Passively disregard everyday thoughts that come to mind, and return to your repetition. Below you will find a detailed, step-by-step sequence to get you started. You may use secular words, or religious words or prayers.

Step 1. Pick a focus word or short phrase that's firmly rooted in your belief system.

Step 2. Sit quietly in a comfortable position.

Step 3. Close your eyes.

Step 4. Relax your muscles.

Step 5. Breathe slowly and naturally, and as you do, repeat your focus word, phrase, or prayer silently to yourself as you exhale.

Step 6. Assume a passive attitude. Don't worry about how well you are doing. When other thoughts come to mind, simply say to yourself, "Oh well," and gently return to the repetition.

Step 7. Continue for ten to twenty minutes.

Step 8. Do not stand immediately. Continue sitting quietly for a minute or so, allowing other thoughts to return. Then open your eyes and sit for another minute before rising.

Step 9. Practice this technique once or twice daily.

Mindfulness and meditation are wonderful tools that can be used almost anywhere. They can prepare your mind to look at and respond to stressful situations as more of an observer instead of as a victim in the circumstances. What really is unique about them is that they can prepare you and give you a glimpse of what it will feel like when you receive a massage. Let's now look at something that is exciting, yet calming—what the world needs more of and its many benefits: Massage!

Chapter 5
What is a Therapeutic Body Massage?

What is a Massage?

You may be surprised, but massage is something we naturally do every day. Have you ever reached up and rubbed your aching neck? When we accidently bump into an object hard enough to cause pain, we instantly reach toward it, apply our hands to the injured area, and rub it.

Whenever an injury occurs to our body, our natural instinct is to ease our aches and pains with our hands. Massage, bodywork, and somatic therapies are defined as the application of various techniques to the muscular structure and soft tissues of the human body.

Massage has been around for centuries. There are paintings in some of the tombs in Egypt, showing massage being used beneficially for the body. However, the Chinese were among the first to recognize its healing value at around 3000 BC. Other cultures, such as the Hindus, Persians, and the Egyptians, have understood the healing power of touch for thousands of years. Hippocrates wrote papers recommending the use of rubbing and friction for joint and circulatory problems.

When we touch or are being touched, its action represents a basic instinct within us. Touch is a potent and extremely useful tool that brings to our awareness what's going on with us and within us. Massage as a form of touch has the potential and can, when administered intentionally and correctly, bring about relaxation and stimulation. Massage also brings comfort and soothes, showing caring and empathy. Another benefit is its ability to relieve stress, anxiety, and depression. It alleviates pain, relieves systems of minor illnesses, and improves emotional and physical well-being.

Although I am a professional Massage Therapist, I have trained individuals to massage others, and I truly believe that anyone can learn how to do it. What is especially beautiful about massage is when you give, you receive. It makes the person receiving feel good and the person giving feel good. Massage affects more than just what is felt at the skin and muscular level. Massage also mediates how we organize our past, experience our present, and anticipate our future. In the next four sections, we will explore together what is happening externally and internally when we receive a massage.

What are the Physical Benefits of Massage?

During a massage, relaxation is accompanied by slower and deeper breathing, causing you to use less energy. Slower and deeper breathing is one of the first indications that a client is beginning to relax. Massage can improve the flow of blood, which helps with poor circulation. Improvement in circulation helps bring a good supply of oxygen and nutrients to the bones. One of the benefits that is obvious to most, is how our muscles respond to massage. During a massage, certain movements relax and stretch our muscles. The reduction of tension and cramps in our muscles is another beneficial result of massage.

The movement of waste in the digestive system increases, and other waste products find their way by means of the bloodstream to the kidneys, where they may be filtered out and eliminated. One technique, tapotement (an energetic modality), may relieve lethargy and fatigue.

Gentle forms of massage have the ability to stimulate the lymphatic system, aiding in the removal of excess waste products. Massage has helped relieve pains that are associated with women's menstrual cycles and symptoms that are related to menopause. Are you beginning to see how effective massage can be? There is more.

What are the Chemical and Mental Benefits of Massage?

Massage therapy offers a number of mood-enhancing benefits because of the body's production and regulation of neurohormones. Research conducted by the Touch Research Institute at the University of Miami revealed that massage increases the availability of all neurohormones affecting brain chemistry.

Dopamine, a neurohormone released by the hypothalamus, is elevated when you are massaged. Dopamine influences fine motor skills like painting or playing a musical instrument. It affects intuition, inspiration, joy, and enthusiasm. Those who exhibit clumsiness and poor focus and who are easily distracted more than likely have a low dopamine level.

The increase of serotonin, a neurohormone activated by massage, regulates emotional behavior, suppresses irritability, and craving for food. If you have a low serotonin level, it is possible you have problems sleeping and may suffer from depression and obsessive-compulsive disorders.

There are other positive results that can be achieved by massage. For example, a 15-minute seated chair massage can elevate epinephrine (adrenaline) levels by stimulating sympathetic nervous system. This can increase a person's alertness. On the other hand, a deeper, slower, longer, and rhythmic massage can reduce epinephrine levels, creating a feeling of relaxation and facilitating deep sleep.

Acupressure and trigger point therapy (applying pressure to tender muscle tissue to relieve pain and dysfunction) are massage techniques that create endorphins, which are compounds known to reduce pain and produce a sense of euphoria.

Oxytocin produced by massage therapy is another neurohormone. It supports feelings of attachment and can help during pregnancy, birthing, and lactation. Massage therapy has also shown to reduce levels of cortisol—the stress-related neurohormone produced by the adrenal glands. Finally, by encouraging sleep, massage can increase the availability of growth hormones, which promote cell division, and is involved in tissue repair, regeneration, and healing.

What are the Spiritual Benefits of Massage?

What is the final conquest? What is it that we are trying to capture? Heroes or heroines in the past set out to conquer a city or country. Some of these fearless heroes rescued princesses. Characters in some of the great adventure stories of the past recovered a magical jewel or sword that would give them unlimited power. The attempt to gain something that will transform us or rescue us is played out in our present life as we are subjected to stress and look for some relief.

The elements in these examples are in most cases symbolic to a larger truth. Figuratively, they are looking for those objects or in the case of the princess, a person, but what they are really looking for is Spirit. This Spirit is not the religious doctrine or dogma. The symbolism of the object or person represents what the hero or heroine is really looking for: the Spirit that allows them to see beyond their immediate reality or circumstance. They are really searching for enlightenment, which will come through a revelation as they discern the ultimate purpose of their challenge. They come to the knowledge that there is more than meets the eyes. What is this more?

In Christianity, it is represented by the verse, "And the Word was made flesh." In Hindu mythology, enlightenment is represented by the union of Siva (universal male form and energy), and in Buddhism it is the union of Yang (male) and Yin (female). What the hero or heroine now realizes, or revels in, is that God is One. He is the unity of male and female. He does not feel separate anymore but feels the "peace that surpasseth all understanding" in Christianity, the "Supreme Bliss" of Hinduism, and Buddhist state of "Nirvana."

During or after their massage, my clients sometimes say, "I feel like I am in heaven," "I have never felt like this before," or, "I feel so peaceful, I don't want to leave this room." I have experienced this on a number of occasions when receiving a massage. We try to articulate the feeling, but you will have to experience it to understand what we are trying to put into words. In this process, as we are being healed, we move past the enlightenment stage of forgiveness toward the emergence of compassion for oneself and for others.

In this state, pain and suffering are suspended—they are not weighing on us. We enter the light, hope, and gift of compassion. Compassion is the peace we all long for. Compassion is the discovery of our **connectedness** to all we have encountered along the way—those who have helped us and those who may have harmed us as well. Compassion is the realization that we are all on this journey and need healing in some area of our lives.

There will always be stressful encounters and situations as we travel on our journey. The spirit of compassion gives us a sense or feeling that we can answer the next stressful event that takes place in our life. When we work with the body and mind, an attitude of **grace** toward self and others emerges. This feeling of compassion that is experienced when you are giving or receiving a massage cannot be reasoned away. This experience is not intellectual, philosophical, or something to be agreed to. Massage is a living experience. Massage is healing, entrancing, and powerful.

Get a Massage! Your Spirit Will Never be the Same!

Massage therapy is a very powerful tool when included in your health care plan when combating stress and when managing it. Research continues to show that massage has a profound effect on the human body when it comes to alleviating and managing stress. The medical community actively embraces therapeutic massage. Many hospitals incorporate onsite massage therapists. As I write, I have a practice at one of the local hospitals.

Seeking out a Licensed Massage Therapist and receiving a massage can be the beginning of you taking charge of your personal health. Making plans to receive massages on a regular basis can do a lot for you and your health. You will feel better about your health and will feel young at heart. Making an investment in your health by getting massages will be a huge return on your setting aside the funds for it. Make massage a part of your wellness plan. Find a Licensed Therapeutic Massage Therapist, set up an appointment, and allow him or her to set up a treatment plan for you.

Massage: It feels good and is good for you.

Win! Win! Win!

Chapter 6
Where Do I Start?

How to Find a Licensed Massage Therapist

After reading about massage therapy and realizing the benefits, you may have decided that you want to take the plunge and try it. The next questions that may enter your mind could include: "Where do I find a massage therapist?" or "What type of massage do I need?" "Will it be a man or a woman that gives me the massage?" "How much will it cost?" "How often should I receive one? I just don't know where to start or what to expect."

All these are good and legitimate questions. In fact, these are just a few of the very same questions that I pondered before I received my very first professional massage. Although today I am a professional massage therapist and have received many massages, questions continue to come up even today if I try some new modality (style of massage) that I have not experienced before.

To begin your search, first I recommend that you check your local directory to see if there are any licensed massage therapy training schools in your local area. You may ask yourself, why can't I just look in the local area business directory book or check the Internet for a massage therapy business? To put it mildly, there are a few wolves, or unlicensed people, in sheep's clothing, masquerading as licensed therapists out there. The second good reason to contact these schools is that they usually supply the local area businesses with massage therapists who work in private practice, hotels, resorts, spas, gyms and, yes, even the YMCA/YWCA. The third reason that I feel is a plus for calling them is that they offer massages at a discounted price given by their students in training at the school. This can be fun, as the students are nervous and so are you.

Jokes aside, what you can really appreciate about the massage schools' clinical is the level of safety that is provided. The students have a supervisor who guides them through the complete process, from the initial interview through the checking on the student periodically to see how your massage is going. Supervisors typically watch the student conclude the massage. This process can be educational for first-time recipients.

The students begin by learning Swedish massage, which is a lighter massage. After learning Swedish, they move on to training in Deep Tissue massage. This process allows you to have the opportunity to take a journey with your therapist. I sometimes visit the schools in my local area for these discounted massages. If you prefer to go to an already licensed massage professional, continue to read the following suggestions. They will include not only using schools as a resource, but they will also help you with your search for a licensed massage professional.

Once you find a massage therapy training school, give them a call, and ask to speak to their program director or the person, or people, who run or supervise their massage training programs clinic. Once you have them on the phone, ask them whether they can recommend a licensed massage therapist in the local area? Normally, the next questions you are asked will be what type of massage you are looking for, or what is going on with your body.

Now, I know you must be thinking, "I don't know anything about the different types of massages." You may not know about the different massages that are offered, but you do know how your body feels. So you tell them, "I am stressed out and just need a relaxing massage." That's it! With that information, the representative from the massage therapy school will most likely be able to point you in the right direction.

If there is not a massage therapy school in your immediate area, check your local area or go online to find listings for Licensed Massaged Therapy Practices. Once you find a few listings, give them a call. A call can save you time, money, and stress. Since the theme of this book is about stress relief and stress management, you are looking for someone who is experienced in relaxation massages. Look and follow the list of questions below. These questions will help you select a massage professional who can provide the type of treatment that you need. Ask your potential therapist these questions:

1. Are you licensed or certified in *your state*?

2. Do you have liability insurance?

3. What increments of time do you offer for massages? 30, 60, 90 minutes?

4. Where are you located? This is a very good question to discover whether they are in a business building or work out of their home.

5.   How long have you been licensed and practicing massage?

6.   What other techniques are you certified in?

7.   Have you taken any classes directly related to the treatment of stress?

8.   After my massage, will you have some information that will help me with daily stress?

9.   Do I have to take off all of my clothes?

These questions are just to give you an idea of how to ask probing questions that will help you make a decision when selecting a massage therapist. Other resources include newspaper ads, a chiropractor, or a primary doctor. Referrals from a friend or an associate who have had experience with a massage therapist can also be a good resource when looking for a well-trained licensed therapist.

Feel free to add any more to this list that will help you in your decision.

What to Expect Before, During, and After Your Massage

Once you have located a licensed massage therapy establishment, your next step is to call and set up an appointment day and time to receive your massage. When you call, you may request a male or female. Once you meet your massage therapist and get past the normal introduction process, he will normally ask you to fill out an intake form. This form will get some of your basic background as it pertains to your body such as:

• How is your general health?

- Is there anything that you are allergic to?

- Is there any particular area you want to be worked on or not worked on?

- Have you had a massage before?

- How would you like to feel when your massage is over?

It is very important that you share with your therapist any health problems or challenges that you are having, or have experienced in the past, when talking about your body. You should also inform your massage therapist of any medications that you are taking.

If you are under a doctor's care, the therapist may require a recommendation or approval from your doctor. These are just a few examples of some of the questions that are on the intake form. These questions help the therapist make an assessment, which will aid him or her in your treatment plan.

Once the intake form is completed, and you discuss why you are there, the therapist should explain the treatment plan to you. This includes the type of massage that you will receive, the general amount of pressure during the massage, and the expected outcome.

The therapist will also tell you the time increments offered. Many people prefer a 60- to 90-minute session for the most advantageous conditions to relax. He will ask you whether you would like to be clothed or unclothed during the massage session.

If you decide to be clothed during your first session, a massage chair or a massage table can be used. Wear comfortable clothing. If you decide to be unclothed, the therapist will direct you to a room for the massage. The room will normally be warm and inviting and have soft music playing to help relax you. It will have a massage table with sheets and blankets on it. The massage therapist will let you know whether your session will begin face up or face down. He will explain to you how to get onto the table for your treatment and then will leave the room.

After he leaves, you will undress to your level of comfort and slide underneath the sheets or blankets. During the massage session, you will be properly draped at all times, with only the area being worked on exposed. The areas being worked on will consist of the ones discussed with your therapist when your treatment plan was discussed.

If your treatment plan calls for a full body massage, it would typically include your back, neck, arms, hands, legs, feet, shoulders, and head. Your therapist should not massage your genitals or breasts, whether you are male or female.

What you will find so interesting about a massage is its potential for personalization. Your treatment plan and session is designed specifically for you. No two people are alike and no two massages are identical. The treatment administered is a culmination of different strokes, different pressures, rubbing rates, and can include body movements such as stretching.

In general, a Swedish-style massage with light or firm strokes is given to calm your nervous system and relax exterior muscle tension. As your body and mind begin to relax, varying pressure will be used in specific areas, continuing to relieve tensions that produce stress. Oils or lotions are applied to the skin in order to reduce excessive friction, which may cause discomfort because of the continuous rubbing that takes place during a massage treatment.

During the massage, just relax and just let go. Most people close their eyes, communicating only if something needs to be changed, such as the temperature of the table or the amount of pressure the therapist is applying. The massage therapist will move relevant parts of the body he is working on. In some cases, he may ask you to assist him with the movement of some part of your body or to roll over.

The beauty and benefit of this stress reliever is that you do not have to do anything once you are on the massage table but receive. Massage is one of the passive solutions to stress, requiring no drugs, pills, alcohol, or strenuous exertion on the part of the person receiving a relaxation massage.

Over the years, some of the comments that I have received from my clients after receiving their massage include, "Herbert, I have never felt so relaxed," "I feel so at peace," "I feel as though I am in Heaven," "I wish that I could feel like this all the time," "I wish that I could remain in this room", and "I just feel so good." These are just a few of the comments that my clients offer, which should give you an idea of what to expect when you receive your massage.

In closing, this book's primary purpose is to explain and show you what stress is and the damage that an inordinate amount of it causes to the body physically, chemically, and mentally. I followed with a source of relief and the management of excessive stress through the healing profession of therapeutic massage. I also presented ways that you can calm your mind and have a feeling and experience similar to the one you have when receiving a massage.

After I spent 22 successful years in the telecommunications field, my career path changed. I am now a professional massage practitioner. God has allowed, and is presently allowing me, to touch my fellow man through massage and to facilitate a physical, chemical, mental, and spiritual change in them that promotes health and well being.

I love what I do, and I am so blessed to be able to do what I do. Massage has changed me and my life, and this extends to my immediate family and beyond. I am more compassionate, which allows the daily growth of feeling connected to the whole to be a reality to me. I want to thank you for reading my book. Now go out and de-stress—get yourself a massage and relax.

Appendix A
Autogenic Relaxation Training

This training exercise was developed in Germany in the early 20th century by two psychologists, Dr. Johannes H. Shultz and Dr. Wolfgang Luthe. This technique will relax the whole body. It's very simple and easy to learn. Begin by finding a comfortable chair to sit upright in. You could practice this technique while lying down, but there is a possibility you may fall asleep. Also, there are steps within it that call for a sitting position.

This technique is for relaxation. Once you finish this exercise, you may want to go to sleep. You may want to try it in helping you fall asleep at bedtime. It is reported that this exercise can help you with insomnia. I use this exercise and it works like magic. You will get more quality rest in a shorter sleep time, and you will have more awake time to be alive and be optimistic about life.

You can have someone to read these words to you until you learn the phrases. You can also record them in your own voice and play them back to yourself until you begin to memorize these simple phrases. Remember it's called autogenic; "auto" means self.

Before you begin:

Now that you are sitting up in your comfortable chair, rest your back against the chair and allow your spine to align, balancing your shoulders. Keep your head upright, without causing any strain. Allow your hands to rest on your lap. Remain comfortably balanced and upright without any physical stress. This exercise normally takes only 20 to 30 minutes.

Begin:

Allow your eyes to slowly close. When you close your eyes, approximately 80% of your sensory input is decreased, making it easier to relax. This starts the relaxation process. Become aware of your breathing. Let it flow in and out effortlessly. Remember, this is only the beginning.

You may feel a small amount of anxiety and apprehension. This is perfectly normal. I can recall the first time I tried this exercise, and I felt that way too. But now I do it with ease, and it seems so natural. Just accept what is going on in your head, because you know that each step that you take will bring you closer to perfect peace and that calm that you are searching for.

Now, take a deep breath...inhale...hold it for three seconds...now let it out completely, feeling all the tension and stress flowing out of the body as you exhale. Do these once again...deep breaths...hold it...1...2...3...exhale completely...all stress flowing out onto the floor. Now, just breathe normally as we begin this autogenic training.

Begin by being aware of your *right foot*. Become completely and totally aware of your *right foot* as part of your body. Now, for just a moment, tense and contract the muscles of this foot ... squeeze ... 1 ... 2 ... 3 ... now relax! Feel the sensation of "letting go" into a deep state of relaxation. Now, place this foot into an even deeper state of relaxation, repeat this phrase silently to yourself...

"My foot is relaxed...

I am relaxed...

I am at peace with my body."

Now move your awareness to your *left foot.* Become completely aware of your left foot as a part of your body. Now, for just a moment, tense and contract the muscles of this *foot* ... squeeze ... 1 ... 2 ... 3 ... now relax! Notice how much better it feels to be relaxed rather than tense. Now, to place this foot into an even deeper state of relaxation, repeat this phrase...silently...to yourself...

"My foot is relaxed...

I am relaxed...

I am at peace with my body."

Now, feel this warm, comfortable feeling move to your ankle ... to your legs ... to your hips. Feel your ankles, legs, and hips becoming *warm ... heavy ... comfortable.* Now, for just a moment, tense and contract the muscles of the legs ... squeeze ... 1 ... 2 ... 3 ... now relax! Feel that sensation of letting go into a deep relaxation. Now, to place this area of your body into a deep state of relaxation, affirm silently to yourself....

"My legs are relaxed...

I am relaxed...

I am at peace with my body."

Now, allow this warm, relaxed feeling to move into your stomach...and into your chest, internally, and affirm to yourself...

"I feel quite quiet...

I am at peace with my inner self."

Now, become aware of all your internal organs and glands, all of the wonderful working parts of your body...and see them all functioning in a calm, relaxed, efficient manner...and again affirm to yourself...

"I feel quite quiet...

I am calm...serene...relaxed."

Now, very gently allow this warm, relaxed feeling to move into your shoulders...then slowly down into your back...feel the upper back relax...the lower back relax...and affirm to yourself...

"My back is relaxed...

I am relaxed.

I am at peace with my inner self."

Feel this warm, comfortable feeling move now into your arms and hands. For just a moment now, very gently tense and contract the muscle of your hands and arms...squeeze...1...2...3...now relax! Feel the sensation of letting go into an even deeper state of relaxation...and now silently affirm...

"My arms and hands are relaxed...

I am relaxed...

I am at peace with my inner self."

Now, feel this warm and comfortable feeling move into your neck...and into your scalp...feel all the tiny muscles of your scalp gently letting go and relaxing...imagine soft, well-trained fingers gently massaging your scalp as you become more and more relaxed.

Feel this warm, relaxed feeling move down into your forehead...feel the forehead becoming smooth and relaxed...the eyebrows relax...the eyes relax...the nose...the cheeks relax...the ears relax...the chin relax...and finally, release any tension that might be centered around the jaw...allow your jaw to relax...to let go...now affirm silently to yourself...

"My face is relaxed...

I am relaxed...

I am at with my inner self."

Now become aware of your entire body...from the tip of your toes to the top of your head...and affirm silently...

"My whole body feels warm...heavy...

comfortable...and relaxed...

I withdraw from thoughts from the surroundings,

And I am serene and still...

I am alert in an easy...calm...

Inward-turned way...

My mind is quiet...and at ease."

And then once again...

"My whole body feels warm...heavy...

comfortable...and relaxed...

I withdraw my thoughts from the surroundings,

And I am serene and still...

I am alert in an easy...calm...

Inward-turned way...

My mind is quiet...and at ease."

Now just sit quietly with yourself for a couple of minutes and then begin to allow your eyes to drift open. Very slowly, open your eyes...then sit quietly for another few moments with your eyes open...Now you can move and stretch...

The autogenic exercise works when you practice it and each time you practice it, you will become a little more relaxed, a little more in control, and another layer of stress will be removed. Stress-less will become second nature to you. Peace and calm will become a habitual state of mind.

Practice this exercise at least once a day for the next 7 to 14 days (twice a day is twice as good). You will be amazed how aware you are and how you begin to view situations. You will feel a sense of power and control over your emotional state.

Appendix B
Long Form Meditation

You can record the following meditation yourself, or ask a friend to speak the words in this meditation in a gentle, calming voice. You can have some relaxing and soft music playing in the background. Where you see the word pause, stop for 15 to 60 seconds or even longer to experience the image fully. Remember, there are no right or wrong ways of doing these visualizations.

Meditation:

Begin by taking some deep breaths. Breathe in peace. Breathe out conflicts and thoughts of fears. Just fill a balloon with them and let go. And when you are ready, look up and let your eyes close gently if they have not by now. And now, let a wave of peace move down through your body. You might give it a color if you like, or repeat a word like "peace" or "relax" to yourself. Let go of the tension in your jaw muscles and your neck and shoulder muscles.

I'd like you to remember sitting in a schoolroom, a classroom with desks. You hear the sound of your classmates around you. The teacher is at the blackboard, filling the board. Do that now. Clean your slate and erase the blackboard of your mind so that you are ready for new lessons and new experiences.

Once you've prepared the slate for new images, words, and lessons, we'll go on a journey. You know where we are headed. We are headed for the middle of nowhere, to your corner of the universe, your own special place in the middle of nowhere, with its vivid colors, textures, aromas, and sound.

Take yourself to that very special place you have created for yourself. Once you arrive there, find a quiet place where you can feel safe and calm. And take a moment here to absorb the pleasant energy of the earth, and the sky, and to take the time for self-healing.

Whatever the problem that you are aware of at this present moment, see yourself eliminating that problem, with whatever treatment or technique that you would feel comfortable utilizing. And now take another moment for yourself, here in this special, safe place that you have chosen and have the knowledge of its secret location.

{Pause}

And when you are done, I'd like you to follow my voice again and dress yourself for work. We are going to build a bridge from your special place to ours, a bridge over a river that will connect with your path through the universe.

So dress for work and be aware of the weave and fabric and texture of your life, and how that has prepared you for your journey. And if your clothing needs to be repaired, repair them with love so that you are prepared for your journey and are dressed appropriately to work on your bridge.

Now take a look at the bridge you have built as you walk across it: how wide, how long, and how strong? What kind of a connection do you have with the universe?

{Pause}

As you cross the bridge to start down your path to begin your wonderful journey, all of the people in your life will be present—family, friends, co-workers, people you have all kinds of relationships with. Stop and touch them, and talk to them. See what changes occur in your feelings and theirs as you all come together. All feelings are appropriate. They are only feelings.

{Pause}

When you have completed that, continue on your path. But if you need to stay, you can catch up with us later. As you walk down the path, you will see an old house off to the side with a garden and a porch. Walk through the garden, up to the porch steps, and into the house and find the living room. And when you find the living room, look around in it for a chest.

Be aware if the chest is in some dusty old corner, or out in an important place. Have you looked at it many times before? When you find your chest, open it and see what lies within, what your heart would like to tell you. What gift or message does your heart have for you as you look inside your chest?

{Pause}

When you find the message within your chest, make it part of you and then come out onto the porch and back to the garden. Find a place where you'd like to plant a seed to create more beauty. And prepare the soil, take the seed and plant it. And then become that seed, sitting in the dark, paying attention to what it feels like to be that seed. Do you know which way to grow? Do you know which way is up? Which way to put down roots? You can't see here in the dark, but you can feel and you can know.

{Pause}

So put down roots to give yourself the nourishment and strength you need to get a grip on things. And then grow, pushing aside problems and obstacles until you break out into the sunlight and then stretch your limbs to the sky. Grow and bloom and blossom. Become that unique, beautiful individual that you already are. And just feel the velvety petal, the aroma, the beautiful color. Grow and blossom where you are.

When you are done, make that flower a part of you. And then continue on your journey. You will come to a quiet, safe place, now stretch out, or sit, and become small enough to enter your body. Go through your body, opening every cell to light, to love. As your organs harmonize, listen to what they have to tell you. Go through your body, repairing, rebuilding, recreating. Walk the corridors of your mind and brain, opening doors, cleaning the shelves of old materials, turning the valves and switches in the different rooms to create the changes that you want to create in your body, so that you create a new self, a new you, a new I.

Then look in the mirror at this new self, this new creation. And look out of the mirror at yourself. Reflect upon what you see, and embrace yourself, accept yourself. Become one with your new self. And then gradually let this new self come back to the room, back to your breathing. Breathe in peace and alertness. Come back gradually, awake and alert, yet relaxed and at peace, back to an awareness of your chair, or the floor. And when the music and the voices have stopped, come back to the room and open your new eyes when you are ready.

Appendix C
More Healthful Massage Benefits

Benefits of Massage

Experts estimate that upwards of 90% of disease is stress-related. And perhaps nothing ages us faster, internally and externally, than high stress. Massage is an effective tool for managing this stress, which translates into:

1. Decreased anxiety
2. Enhanced sleep quality
3. Greater energy
4. Improved concentration
5. Increased circulation
6. Reduced fatigue

Massage can also specifically help address a number of health issues. Bodywork can:

1. Alleviate *lower back pain* and improve range of motion. Assist with shorter, easier labor for *expectant mothers* and shorten maternity hospital stays.

2. Ease *medication dependence*.

3. Enhance *immunity* by stimulating lymph flow—the body's natural defense system.

4. Exercise and stretch *weak, tight, or atrophied muscles*.

5. Help *athletes* of any level prepare for, and recover from, strenuous workouts.

6. Improve the condition of the body's largest organ—the skin.

7. Increase *joint flexibility*.

8. Lessen *depression and anxiety*.

9. Promote tissue regeneration, reducing *scar tissue and stretch marks*.

10. Pump oxygen and nutrients into tissues and vital organs, improving *circulation*.

11. Reduce *post-surgery adhesions and swelling*.

12. Reduce *spasms and cramping*.

13. Relax and soften injured, tired, and *overused muscles*.

14. Release endorphins—amino acids that work as the body's natural *painkiller*.

15. Relieve *migraine* pain.

Testimonials

As a result of getting a massage, I no longer experience tension headaches. I am greatly refreshed and perform better at my job, and I feel very supported by my workplace that allows this service to come into my workplace. I cannot say enough about the good things that result—including my state of mind!

Specifically, I enjoy feeling the muscle tension leave, and enjoy the transition from uptight and tense—to relaxed and calm. Three other benefits I receive from massage are:

- A time to clear my head and relax that I would not otherwise allow myself
- It lowers my blood pressure
- It's the only time in my week that someone else is attending to me! (As a mom, I do the attending to!)

I would *highly* recommend this service to someone else—everyone else! It is so important for us to stop in the middle of a busy, stressful work day (or work week) to relax and take care of ourselves. It helps to keep us from getting sick, helps to keep us from getting burned out at work, and helps us to focus better on our tasks when we are taking care of ourselves. To me, a massage every other week is as important to me as exercise and eating right!

I want to add that Mr. Gooden is the best massage therapist that I've ever had! He has a kind and peaceful manner, and is very skilled at massage. He is always professional, always keeps appointments, and is a very caring individual. I would *highly* recommend Mr. Gooden to everyone I know—and already do that here at Children's of Alabama!

—Michelle J.

The massage relaxes me and gives me a restart for the day. It really improves productivity for the afternoon. I enjoy the down time and clearing of my mind the most. Convenient location, price, reduces tension, and stress. Yes, it's very effective, the environment is private, and the services are professional. I enjoy this benefit and wish this could be offered more than once a week.

—Kim S.

I have been enjoying the massage services of Herbert Gooden for several years now. Not only does Herbert excel in his massage techniques, he listens to your concerns and needs, and he seeks to provide the type of massage you need in the most professional manner.

At the end of the massage session, you feel rejuvenated, ready to face your next task with an abundance of strength and energy. Herbert has brought back that balance—your body is relaxed as well as your mind, and it touches your spirit. There is an art to those healing hands.

Experience this for yourself, you won't be disappointed.

—Frank H.

Herbert has helped me in so many ways over the years and especially in the last 18 months, when I have been seeing him on a weekly or biweekly basis.

The stress my body feels from working at the desk for long hours is relieved when he does the deep tissue massage and targets areas that need special attention. I know now that regularly seeing him has made the pain so much less for me, and I look forward to seeing him.

He also has shown me techniques to try at home, such as relaxation techniques, stretching techniques, and ideas to get in a little exercise while I am at work. Working with Herbert has truly made a difference in my life.

—Lynn B.

Thank you for helping me! I had never received a massage before because I always thought it was a luxury that I could not afford. The massage has allowed me to help lessen the pain that I am experiencing. I enjoyed the calming atmosphere and vast knowledge and experience of the therapist.

Benefits include a feeling of well being; the knowledge that I am complementing chiropractic treatments with massage for a better overall effect; and relaxation, stress relief, and calmness. I would wholeheartedly recommend Herbert and his healing hands. He is a gentleman with a talent for putting you at ease, and he is very knowledgeable, informative, and helpful.

Thank you for helping me.

—Bonnie B.

When I receive a massage, it puts me in a relaxed mood and decreases my stress. I most enjoy the face, head, and neck massage. I also really love the ambiance, and Herbert has a calming demeanor. He is always pleasant.

Other benefits from massage are less tension, moodiness, and irritability. I would definitely recommend getting a massage for others. I wish I could give my staff massages for staff appreciation.

Herbert is the best! He is very thorough, attentive, and very professional. I have been to a lot of massage therapists, and he is one of the best I've had.

—Ehrica S.

I used to suffer from debilitating stress headaches and as a working mother, I found it nearly impossible to work a massage into my schedule. When on-site massage therapy was deployed by Children's as part of our ongoing stress management and wellness strategy, having access to massage therapy at work was a perfect solution to my scheduling dilemma.

I find Herbert to be a calm, spiritual, positive, and wellness-focused therapist whose massages are technically superior. The ability to have his level of competence and service without having to drive somewhere before or after work or on the weekends is such a blessing. I recommend him highly.

—Sandy T.

Onsite massage has allowed me to take advantage of a low-cost alternative therapy and is such a convenience being here at work. I am now receiving pain relief for a medically diagnosed condition. I enjoy all that it has to offer—the aromatherapy and the relaxing music, combined with deep tissue massage. It is a great experience and outcome for me.

I have a greater appreciation for the effectiveness of non-conventional treatment such as massage therapy. I now have a means of relaxation during an often stressful workday and am able to walk pain-free.

I highly recommend massage therapy as an effective means to treat joint conditions, and to control and alleviate joint and muscle pain.

Thank you so much! I wished more healthcare professionals recognized the medical benefits of massage therapy as an option rather than depending on conventional medications to treat symptoms.

—Susan T.

www.ingramcontent.com/pod-product-compliance
Lightning Source LLC
Chambersburg PA
CBHW070816290526
45795CB00002B/729